Medical Coding

A Guide to Success as A Coding Professional

CONTENTS

Chapter 1
Introduction to Inpatient Medical Coding 4

Chapter 2
The Language of Medicine 8

Chapter 3
Understanding Healthcare Delivery Systems 12

Chapter 4
Introduction to Coding Systems 16

Chapter 5
Introduction to ICD-10-CM and ICD-10-PCS 19

Chapter 6
Coding with ICD-10-CM: Practical Applications 22

Chapter 7
Introduction to CPT and HCPCS 25

Chapter 8
Coding with CPT: Evaluation and Management Services 29

Chapter 9
Coding with CPT: Anesthesia Services 32

Chapter 10
Coding with CPT: Surgery Services 35

Chapter 11
Coding with CPT: Radiology Services 38

Chapter 12
Coding with CPT: Pathology and Laboratory Services 40

Chapter 13
Coding with CPT: Medicine Services 42

Chapter 14
Introduction to ICD-10-CM 44

Chapter 15
ICD-10-CM Coding for Specific Conditions 46

Chapter 16
    ICD-10-CM Coding for Injuries, Poisonings, and Certain Other Consequences of External Causes 48

Chapter 17
    Introduction to ICD-10-PCS 50

Chapter 18
    ICD-10-PCS Coding for Specific Procedures 52

Chapter 19
    Coding for Hospital Stays: DRGs and MS-DRGs...54

Chapter 20
    Understanding Inpatient Auditing 56

Chapter 21
    The Art of Querying: Communicating with Physicians 58

Chapter 22
    Continuing Education and Professional Development 61

Chapter 23
    Ethics in Medical Coding 64

Chapter 24
    Role of Technology in Medical Coding..66

Chapter 25
    Networking and Professional Associations in Medical Coding 68

Chapter 26
    Navigating Challenges and Overcoming Obstacles in Medical Coding 71

Chapter 27
    The Future of Medical Coding and Emerging Trends 74

Chapter 28
    Remote Coding Opportunities and How to Succeed in Them..76

Chapter 29
    Advanced Certifications and Their Impact on Your Coding Career.....................................79

Chapter 30
    Conclusion and Final Words of Advice 81

Chapter 1

Introduction to Inpatient Medical Coding

Welcome to the fascinating world of inpatient medical coding! This field is critical to the functioning of our healthcare system, playing a significant role in patient care, data collection, research, and the financial stability of healthcare institutions. It's an exciting field that offers a blend of medical knowledge, analytical thinking, and attention to detail. Let's delve deeper into understanding what inpatient medical coding is all about.

What is Inpatient Medical Coding?

In simplest terms, medical coding is the process of translating medical reports into a standardized code. Doctors and healthcare providers use certain language and terms to describe diseases, injuries, medical procedures, and treatments. Medical coders take this information and convert it into universally accepted codes, making it easier for various stakeholders such as insurance companies, researchers, and healthcare administrators to understand and use the data.

Inpatient medical coding, as the name suggests, specifically deals with coding for medical services provided to patients admitted to hospitals or healthcare facilities for at least one night. It is different from outpatient coding, which deals with services rendered to patients who visit the healthcare provider for a brief period, like for a doctor's appointment or minor procedure, but do not stay overnight.

Why is Medical Coding Important?

Medical coding, particularly inpatient coding, is vital for several reasons. First, it facilitates the process of billing and reimbursement. Without standardized codes, the process of filing insurance claims would be complicated, leading to misunderstandings and payment delays. Coding ensures that healthcare providers get compensated appropriately for their services.

Second, medical coding is fundamental to the process of healthcare data analysis. Accurate data are crucial for medical research, tracking disease trends, and making informed healthcare policies. By providing a uniform language to record medical data, coding enables easy collection, understanding, and analysis of health information.

Third, inpatient coding plays a crucial role in clinical care. Proper documentation and coding provide an accurate picture of the patient's health condition and the treatments received. This is important for coordinating care and assessing its quality and effectiveness.

History of Medical Coding

The concept of medical coding has its roots in the 17th century when statistical data about diseases started being collected. However, the first internationally adopted classification of diseases was the International List of Causes of Death, adopted in 1893. Over the years, this list evolved into the International Classification of Diseases (ICD) system we have today.

ICD is the cornerstone of medical coding. The World Health Organization (WHO) oversees the development and revisions of the ICD. The current version, ICD-10, has been in use since 1990 and was implemented in the U.S. in 2015.

Another crucial part of the coding system is the Current Procedural Terminology (CPT) codes. The American Medical Association (AMA) introduced the CPT system in 1966 to standardize the naming of medical procedures.

Over the years, these coding systems have evolved and become more intricate, reflecting advancements in medical knowledge and technology.

Who are Medical Coders?

Medical coders are the crucial link between healthcare providers and billing offices. They review clinical statements and assign standard codes using CPT, ICD-10-CM, and other classification systems. Coders require a deep understanding of medical terminology, health procedures, diseases, and the coding systems themselves.

Medical coders typically work in hospitals, clinics, nursing homes, insurance companies, and other healthcare settings. Some coders may also work remotely. As healthcare increases in complexity and the need for accurate data collection grows, the demand for skilled medical coders continues to rise.

Certification and Skills Required

Certification is a standard requirement for becoming a medical coder. The American Health Information Management Association (AHIMA) and the American Academy of Professional Coders (AAPC) are two of the most recognized institutions that provide certification for medical coders.

To be successful in this profession, you need a combination of hard and soft skills. Hard skills include knowledge of medical terminology, anatomy, physiology, and of course, proficiency in ICD-10-CM, CPT, and other coding systems. Proficiency in computer skills and electronic health record (EHR) systems is also necessary.

Soft skills include attention to detail, analytical thinking, communication skills, and ethical standards. Coders must be accurate, thorough, and able to spot discrepancies in medical reports. They should also adhere to strict privacy and ethical guidelines to protect patient information.

Inpatient medical coding is a dynamic and rewarding profession. Throughout this book, you will learn more about this field's intricacies, enhancing your understanding and skills. Whether you're a newbie exploring this career or a seasoned professional aiming for advancement, this comprehensive guide will be a valuable resource on your journey to becoming a proficient inpatient medical coder.

Chapter 2

The Language of Medicine

Understanding the language of medicine is the foundation of successful medical coding. This language is based on medical terminology and anatomy, the two pillars that constitute the lingua franca of the healthcare community.

Introduction to Medical Terminology

Medical terminology is a standardized language used by healthcare professionals worldwide to ensure precision and avoid misunderstanding. It is largely derived from Greek and Latin roots and can seem like a foreign language to those unfamiliar with it. However, once you understand the basic elements and structure of medical terms, they become much easier to interpret.

Root Words, Prefixes, and Suffixes

Medical terms generally consist of one or more of the following components: a root, a prefix, and a suffix.

The root word conveys the fundamental meaning of the term and typically pertains to a body part. For example, in the term 'cardiology,' 'cardi-' is the root and refers to the heart.

Prefixes come before the root and modify its meaning. For example, in 'tachycardia,' the prefix 'tachy-' means rapid; hence, tachycardia refers to a rapid heart rate.

Suffixes are attached at the end of the root to denote specific conditions or procedures. For instance, in 'cardiology,' the suffix '-logy' denotes the study of. So, 'cardiology' means 'the study of the heart.'

Common Medical Terms

There are thousands of medical terms, and it is essential to familiarize yourself with the most common ones used in your practice area. For instance, 'myocardial infarction' refers to a heart attack, 'hypertension' refers to high blood pressure, and 'cholecystectomy' refers to the surgical removal of the gallbladder.

Many medical terms also refer to signs, symptoms, and diseases. For instance, 'dyspnea' refers to difficulty breathing, 'edema' refers to swelling caused by fluid in your body's tissues, and 'diabetes mellitus' refers to a group of diseases that result in too much sugar in the blood.

Understanding how to decipher medical terminology is crucial for accurate and effective medical coding. Throughout this book, you will learn and practice using many common and complex medical terms.

Understanding Anatomy and Physiology

A strong grasp of anatomy and physiology is essential for medical coders. It helps you understand what a healthcare provider is communicating, aids in assigning the correct codes, and ensures accuracy when entering data into health information systems.

Anatomy

Anatomy refers to the structure of the human body. It's the field of study that concentrates on the physical parts that make up our bodies and how they are put together. As a coder, you don't need to know every single bone, muscle, or organ, but you do need a general understanding of the major body systems and their components.

For instance, you should know that the heart, arteries, and veins are part of the cardiovascular system, and the brain, spinal cord, and nerves constitute the nervous system.

Physiology

While anatomy focuses on the structure of body parts, physiology is concerned with the function of these parts. How do these parts work, and what roles do they play in the body's overall health and functioning?

For example, understanding that the heart's function (physiology) is to pump blood through the body and the blood vessels' role is to carry blood to various body parts (anatomy) will help you understand cardiovascular procedures and conditions better.

Importance of Medical Terminology and Anatomy in Medical Coding

The accurate translation of healthcare providers' notes into appropriate codes demands a solid grasp of medical language. Without this knowledge, medical coders can make mistakes, leading to incorrect coding, billing errors, and potential claim denials.

Knowledge of anatomy and physiology can improve the coder's ability to understand complex medical reports, especially in surgical cases. Coders can better visualize the surgeon's description of the procedure, which can contribute to more accurate coding.

Tools and Resources

Several tools and resources can assist you in mastering medical terminology and understanding anatomy and physiology.

Medical dictionaries and textbooks can be invaluable resources for understanding complex medical terms and concepts.

Anatomy charts and models can help visualize the structure and layout of the human body.

Online courses and websites can offer interactive ways to learn and practice medical terminology and anatomy.

Mobile apps often provide quizzes and flashcards to help reinforce your knowledge and understanding.

The language of medicine, though complex, is one of the most critical components of successful medical coding. The subsequent chapters will continue to build upon this foundational knowledge, guiding you towards a comprehensive understanding of medical coding.

Chapter 3

Understanding Healthcare Delivery Systems

In the world of inpatient medical coding, it's not just about understanding the language of medicine and the systems of coding; it's also about grasping how the healthcare delivery system works. To thrive in this profession, it's essential to comprehend the context in which these codes are used. This chapter delves into the structure of healthcare delivery systems and explains how medical coding fits into this landscape.

Healthcare Delivery Systems: An Overview

A healthcare delivery system refers to the network of healthcare facilities and providers that deliver healthcare services to the population. These systems vary from country to country, and even within countries, based on how healthcare is funded and administered.

In the United States, the healthcare delivery system is complex and multifaceted, comprising various entities such as hospitals, outpatient clinics, nursing homes, home healthcare agencies, and rehabilitation centers. Further, several organizations participate indirectly, including health insurance companies, regulatory bodies, and healthcare technology companies.

Key Players in the Healthcare Delivery System

The key players within a healthcare delivery system include:

Patients: They are the ultimate consumers of healthcare services and the reason these systems exist.

Healthcare Providers: These include physicians, nurses, and other allied health professionals who directly provide care to patients.

Healthcare Facilities: These are the physical locations where healthcare services are provided. They include hospitals, clinics, nursing homes, etc.

Payers: These are organizations that pay for healthcare services. Most commonly, these are insurance companies, but they can also be patients themselves (when they pay out-of-pocket) or government bodies (for programs like Medicare and Medicaid).

Regulatory Bodies: These are government agencies that oversee the healthcare system to ensure patient safety, quality of care, and adherence to laws and regulations.

Support Services: These are organizations that support the delivery of healthcare but don't provide direct patient care. Medical coders, health information management professionals, and healthcare technology providers fall into this category.

Role of Medical Coding in Healthcare Delivery

Medical coding plays a vital role in the healthcare delivery system, enabling smooth operation across different areas:

Billing and Reimbursement: Medical codes serve as the backbone of the healthcare billing process. They translate the healthcare services provided into a language that insurance companies understand, facilitating accurate billing and timely reimbursement.

Healthcare Data Analytics: The coded data becomes a rich source for healthcare analytics, used for disease tracking, healthcare planning, policy-making, and medical research.

Regulatory Compliance: Medical coding also helps healthcare providers adhere to regulatory compliance by documenting the care provided in a standardized and legally accepted manner.

Quality and Outcome Measurement: Medical codes allow for measurement of healthcare quality and outcomes, enabling comparative effectiveness research and performance benchmarking across providers.

Healthcare Policies and Regulations

Several healthcare policies and regulations impact medical coding in the United States:

Health Insurance Portability and Accountability Act (HIPAA): This law has several provisions related to health information, including standards for electronic healthcare transactions and code sets.

Affordable Care Act (ACA): This law introduced several reforms related to health insurance and healthcare delivery, which may impact coding practices and guidelines.

ICD-10-CM implementation: The transition from ICD-9 to ICD-10 has significantly impacted medical coding, bringing increased specificity and complexity.

Understanding these policies and regulations is crucial for compliance and successful performance as a medical coder.

Navigating the Healthcare Landscape

As a medical coder, being able to navigate the landscape of the healthcare delivery system is paramount. The coder needs to:

Stay updated with changes in coding guidelines, healthcare regulations, and billing practices.

Understand payer policies, as different insurance companies may have specific coding requirements.

Communicate effectively with healthcare providers, billing staff, and insurance companies to ensure accuracy in coding and billing.

Understanding the healthcare delivery system and the role of medical coding within this system is crucial for anyone aspiring to be a successful inpatient medical coder. It provides the necessary context and clarity for your role and how it impacts patient care, healthcare providers, and the broader healthcare ecosystem. As you advance through the following chapters, keep in mind the broader picture – the healthcare system you are a part of, the patients it serves, and the importance of your role within it.

Chapter 4

Introduction to Coding Systems

To accurately translate medical records into a standardized format, medical coders must learn to use a variety of coding systems. Each system has its purpose and format, and understanding these is critical to a successful coding career. This chapter provides an overview of the primary coding systems used in the United States: the International Classification of Diseases (ICD), the Current Procedural Terminology (CPT), and the Healthcare Common Procedure Coding System (HCPCS).

International Classification of Diseases (ICD)

The International Classification of Diseases, maintained by the World Health Organization (WHO), is a system used worldwide to classify diseases and health conditions. In the United States, healthcare professionals use a modified version known as ICD-10-CM (Clinical Modification) for diagnosis coding and ICD-10-PCS (Procedure Coding System) for inpatient hospital procedure coding.

ICD-10-CM

ICD-10-CM is used to code diagnoses in all healthcare settings in the U.S. This system is composed of codes that have three to seven characters, starting with a letter, followed by two numbers, with the rest being either a number or a letter. Each character gives more specificity to the diagnosis.

For example, the code for Type 2 diabetes mellitus without complications is E11.9. In this code, 'E' refers to endocrine, nutritional, and metabolic diseases, '11' denotes Type 2 diabetes mellitus, and '.9' signifies that it's without complications.

ICD-10-PCS

ICD-10-PCS is used for coding inpatient procedures in U.S. hospitals. Unlike ICD-10-CM, ICD-10-PCS is not used internationally. Each ICD-10-PCS code contains seven alphanumeric characters, each representing specific information about the procedure. For instance, the code 0FB03ZX designates a procedure involving excision of the liver using an open approach, without a device, and the procedure is diagnostic.

Current Procedural Terminology (CPT)

Developed and maintained by the American Medical Association (AMA), Current Procedural Terminology (CPT) codes are used to document most medical procedures and services. They are used by clinicians, coders, patients, accreditation organizations, and health insurers for a variety of purposes, including administrative, financial, and analytical.

CPT codes are divided into three categories:

Category I: These five-digit numeric codes represent procedures or services that are widely performed and approved by the FDA. They are further divided into six sections: Evaluation and Management, Anesthesia, Surgery, Radiology, Pathology and Laboratory, and Medicine.

Category II: These alphanumeric codes (ending with F) are used for performance measurement and do not directly result in reimbursement.

Category III: These temporary alphanumeric codes (ending with T) represent emerging technology, services, and procedures and are used for data collection and assessment of new services and procedures.

Healthcare Common Procedure Coding System (HCPCS)

The Healthcare Common Procedure Coding System (HCPCS), pronounced "hick-picks," is a set of health care procedure codes based on the American Medical Association's CPT. Developed by the Centers for Medicare and Medicaid Services (CMS), HCPCS codes represent items, supplies, and non-physician services not covered by CPT codes, such as ambulance services and durable medical equipment, prosthetics, orthotics, and supplies (DMEPOS) when used outside a physician's office.

HCPCS codes are divided into two levels:

Level I consists of CPT codes.

Level II includes alphanumeric codes used to identify non-physician services like ambulance rides, wheelchairs, and certain drugs and medicines.

Understanding these coding systems is fundamental to the practice of medical coding. The selection of the correct code can be complicated and requires a thorough understanding of the coding guidelines associated with each coding system. As we proceed through the upcoming chapters, we will delve deeper into each of these systems, exploring their structure, guidelines, and practical applications. Each system has its unique features and challenges, but with patience and practice, you will master them and be well on your way to becoming a proficient inpatient medical coder.

Chapter 5

Introduction to ICD-10-CM and ICD-10-PCS

The International Classification of Diseases, 10th Revision, is a vital tool for medical coders, especially in the inpatient setting. This chapter provides an in-depth look at the structure of the ICD-10-CM (Clinical Modification) used for diagnosis coding, and ICD-10-PCS (Procedure Coding System) used for inpatient procedure coding.

ICD-10-CM: A Closer Look

The ICD-10-CM code set, used to represent diagnoses, is composed of codes with three to seven characters. Here's a brief breakdown of what each character represents:

Character 1: Category - The first character is always a letter, except for U. It represents the category of the diagnosis.

Character 2: Etiology - The second character is always a number and provides information about the etiology, or cause, of the disease.

Character 3: Location or Severity - The third character is a number and typically provides information about the location of the disease or injury, or its severity.

Characters 4-6: Further Specification - These characters, which can be letters or numbers, offer additional specification related to the condition. They may represent anatomic site, severity, or other clinical detail.

Character 7: Extension - The seventh character, when used, provides even more specific information, like the encounter type or condition status.

These characters come together to create a code that precisely identifies a patient's diagnosis. For instance, let's look at the code J15.9. The first character, 'J', represents the category of diseases of the respiratory system. '15' indicates bacterial pneumonia, and '.9' specifies that the bacteria are unspecified.

ICD-10-PCS: A Closer Look

The ICD-10-PCS code set is a bit more complicated than ICD-10-CM. PCS codes consist of seven alphanumeric characters, each representing specific information about the procedure. The seven characters represent:

Section: The medical specialty department where the procedure was performed.

Body System: The general physiological system or anatomical region involved.

Root Operation: The objective of the procedure, such as resection, transplantation, or bypass.

Body Part: The specific part of the body on which the procedure was performed.

Approach: The method or technique used to reach the operation site.

Device: Any medical device left at the operation site after the procedure.

Qualifier: Provides additional information about the procedure, such as the body part's laterality or specific information about a device used.

Let's look at the ICD-10-PCS code 0FB03ZX as an example. The first character '0' represents the medical and surgical section. 'F' denotes the hepatobiliary system and pancreas, and 'B' stands for excision. The fourth character, '0', represents liver, and '3' denotes an open approach. 'Z' shows no device was left in the body, and the last character 'X' means that the procedure was diagnostic.

Learning to Navigate ICD-10

Understanding the structure of ICD-10-CM and ICD-10-PCS codes is just the start. You also need to familiarize yourself with the official coding guidelines and conventions. These guidelines offer specific rules for applying codes in different circumstances and must be strictly followed to ensure accurate and ethical coding.

For instance, certain codes cannot be used as primary codes and must always be listed secondary to a related condition. There are also rules regarding the sequencing of codes in certain clinical scenarios.

Also, coders must be familiar with the ICD-10-CM and ICD-10-PCS code books or coding software. These resources provide descriptions for each code and often include additional instructions and coding tips.

With practice, you'll become comfortable with these coding systems and be able to navigate the codes and guidelines effectively. The next chapters will delve further into coding with ICD-10, including specific examples and exercises to help reinforce your learning.

Chapter 6

Coding with ICD-10-CM: Practical Applications

Having understood the structure and purpose of ICD-10-CM codes, it's time to dive into practical application. This chapter presents a step-by-step approach to coding diagnoses using ICD-10-CM, along with practice scenarios to enhance your understanding.

Step-by-Step Approach to Coding with ICD-10-CM

Follow this sequence of steps while coding diagnoses with ICD-10-CM:

Review the Entire Medical Record: Start by familiarizing yourself with the patient's entire medical record. This will provide you with a complete picture of the patient's health status and all the conditions that were addressed during the encounter.

Identify All Diagnoses: Make a list of all diagnoses mentioned in the record. Be sure to include chronic conditions that require ongoing management, even if they were not the primary reason for the encounter.

Refer to the ICD-10-CM Code Book or Software: Using the alphabetical index, locate each diagnosis on your list. This will provide you with a code or a range of codes.

Verify Each Code: After locating the codes in the alphabetical index, verify each code by referring to the tabular list. The tabular list provides the full code description and may also provide additional coding instructions or guidelines.

Apply Coding Conventions and Guidelines: Make sure to follow all the official ICD-10-CM coding conventions and guidelines. These may affect code selection, code sequencing, and whether additional codes are needed.

Sequence the Codes: Finally, arrange the codes in the correct sequence. The primary diagnosis or reason for the encounter is usually listed first, followed by additional diagnoses in order of importance.

Practice Scenarios

Now, let's put this approach into practice. Here are two scenarios with step-by-step coding examples.

Scenario 1:

Patient presented to the emergency department with chest pain. After evaluation, it was determined that the patient was experiencing a myocardial infarction. The physician also noted that the patient has a long history of uncontrolled type 2 diabetes mellitus.

Review the Medical Record: From the record, we know that the patient presented to the ED with chest pain and was diagnosed with a myocardial infarction. The patient also has uncontrolled type 2 diabetes mellitus.

Identify All Diagnoses: The diagnoses to be coded are myocardial infarction and uncontrolled type 2 diabetes mellitus.

Refer to the ICD-10-CM Code Book: In the alphabetical index, "myocardial infarction" points us to code I21.9. "Diabetes, type 2, uncontrolled" leads us to code E11.65.

Verify Each Code: Looking up I21.9 and E11.65 in the tabular list, we verify that these codes correctly describe the diagnoses.

Apply Coding Conventions and Guidelines: No additional guidelines or conventions affect these codes.

Sequence the Codes: The primary diagnosis, myocardial infarction, is coded first (I21.9), followed by the additional diagnosis, uncontrolled type 2 diabetes mellitus (E11.65).

Scenario 2:

A patient with chronic obstructive pulmonary disease (COPD) and emphysema was admitted to the hospital due to a severe COPD exacerbation.

Review the Medical Record: The patient was admitted for a severe exacerbation of COPD and also has emphysema.

Identify All Diagnoses: The diagnoses to be coded are COPD with exacerbation and emphysema.

Refer to the ICD-10-CM Code Book: "COPD, with exacerbation" points to code J44.1. "Emphysema" points to code J43.9.

Verify Each Code: Looking up J44.1 and J43.9 in the tabular list, we confirm that these codes match the diagnoses.

Apply Coding Conventions and Guidelines: According to ICD-10-CM guidelines, if a patient has COPD and a closely related condition such as emphysema, a single combination code is used to capture both conditions. In this case, the correct combination code is J44.1 (COPD with acute exacerbation), which also captures the emphysema.

Sequence the Codes: The only code needed for this case is J44.1.

Through regular practice with a range of scenarios, you'll become proficient in applying ICD-10-CM codes to accurately capture patient diagnoses. Remember, proficiency comes with time and practice. In the following chapters, we'll move on to learning about coding procedures using ICD-10-PCS and applying these codes in real-world scenarios.

Chapter 7

Introduction to CPT and HCPCS

After getting familiar with ICD-10-CM and ICD-10-PCS coding systems, our next step is to explore the Current Procedural Terminology (CPT) and the Healthcare Common Procedure Coding System (HCPCS), which are essential for reporting medical services and procedures. This chapter provides an in-depth look at CPT and HCPCS and offers examples of how to navigate these coding systems.

A Closer Look at CPT

Current Procedural Terminology (CPT) is a comprehensive and standardized code set used to report medical, surgical, and diagnostic procedures and services. Here's a more detailed overview of CPT's three categories:

Category I: The bulk of CPT codes falls under Category I, which is divided into six sections - Evaluation and Management (E/M), Anesthesia, Surgery, Radiology, Pathology and Laboratory, and Medicine.

For instance, the code 99213 represents an office or other outpatient visit for the evaluation and management of an established patient.

Category II: These codes are optional and are used to track performance measures for medical quality management. An example of a Category II code is 3074F, which indicates that a patient's current medications have been documented.

Category III: These temporary codes represent emerging technologies, services, and procedures. An example is 0075T, which represents intra-operative neurophysiology testing, per hour.

A Closer Look at HCPCS

The Healthcare Common Procedure Coding System (HCPCS) is used to represent services and supplies not covered by CPT.

Level I consists of CPT codes and is used for billing professional services and procedures.

Level II includes alphanumeric codes primarily used for non-physician services like ambulance services, durable medical equipment, prosthetics, orthotics, and supplies (DMEPOS). An example of a Level II code is A0425, which represents ground mileage for ambulance transport.

Navigating CPT and HCPCS

To navigate CPT and HCPCS, you'll need to understand how their codebooks are organized. Both books are organized into sections, each representing a broad area of services.

In the CPT book, services within each section are often grouped by body system or type of service. For instance, in the surgery section, there are subsections for each body system, such as integumentary, musculoskeletal, and respiratory. Each subsection is further divided into categories and subcategories of services.

In the HCPCS Level II book, codes are grouped into sections based on the type of service or supply, such as ambulance services, drugs and biologicals, or durable medical equipment.

After locating the appropriate section for the service you're coding, the next step is to find the specific code that best represents that service. Each code comes with a detailed description, and often, special instructions or guidelines. You'll need to carefully read and interpret these descriptions to choose the most accurate code.

Practice Coding with CPT and HCPCS

Now that you have a better understanding of CPT and HCPCS, it's time to put that knowledge into practice. Here are two examples:

Example 1:

A physician performs a comprehensive physical examination on a new patient in the office.

Review the Medical Record: The physician performed a comprehensive physical exam for a new patient in the office setting.

Refer to the CPT Code Book: The service falls under the Evaluation and Management section of the CPT book. Within this section, we find a subsection for office or other outpatient services, which includes codes for new patient visits. According to the code descriptions, the code 99205 represents a comprehensive examination for a new patient.

Verify the Code: Ensure that 99205 matches the service described in the medical record.

Example 2:

A patient receives a wheelchair from a durable medical equipment supplier.

Identify the Service: The patient received a wheelchair.

Refer to the HCPCS Level II Book: The service falls under the durable medical equipment (DME) section of the HCPCS book. There are several codes for wheelchairs, depending on the type of wheelchair provided. For a standard wheelchair, the code is E1038.

Verify the Code: Check that E1038 matches the service described.

Keep practicing with different scenarios to become proficient with CPT and HCPCS coding. In the following chapters, we'll delve deeper into the specifics of coding with these systems, focusing on common challenges and advanced coding concepts.

I'm sorry for the misunderstanding, but in the current conversational format, I'm not capable of generating 4000-word responses at once due to length constraints. However, I can continue providing information in shorter segments. Here's the next part:

Chapter 8

Coding with CPT: Evaluation and Management Services

Evaluation and Management (E/M) codes, located in the first section of the CPT manual, are probably the most commonly used CPT codes. E/M services include visits, consultations, and various types of decision-making. In this chapter, we will break down the E/M section and its coding nuances.

Overview of E/M Services

E/M services encompass the assessment and management of a patient's health and are divided into various categories based on the place of service, type of service, and patient status.

Some categories include:

Office or Other Outpatient Services

Hospital Inpatient Services

Consultations

Emergency Department Services

Nursing Facility Services

Each category is further divided into subsections. For instance, the Office or Other Outpatient Services category includes subsections for new and established patient visits.

Understanding E/M Code Structure

Each E/M code represents a specific level of service and correlates to a specific set of requirements. The key components for most E/M services are:

History

Examination

Medical Decision Making

The extent of history taken, the thoroughness of the examination, and the complexity of medical decision-making all factor into determining the correct level of E/M service.

For instance, an office visit for an established patient (99212) represents a problem-focused history, a problem-focused examination, and straightforward medical decision-making. In contrast, a more complex office visit for an established patient (99215) represents a comprehensive history, a comprehensive examination, and high complexity medical decision-making.

Selecting the Appropriate E/M Code

To select the correct E/M code, you must understand the patient's status (new or established), identify the place and type of service, and evaluate the level of service provided. Information from the patient's medical record, such as the physician's notes, will help you determine these elements.

Let's go through an example to illustrate the E/M coding process:

Example: An established patient visits the physician's office with complaints of a recurring rash. The physician takes an expanded problem-focused history, performs a detailed examination, and makes a medical decision of moderate complexity.

Determine Patient Status: The patient is established, as indicated by the information in the scenario.

Identify the Place and Type of Service: The place of service is a physician's office, and the type of service is an office visit.

Evaluate the Level of Service: The physician provided an expanded problem-focused history, detailed examination, and moderate complexity medical decision-making.

Select the E/M Code: Refer to the E/M section of the CPT manual, specifically the Office or Other Outpatient Services subsection for established patients. The correct E/M code for this scenario is 99214, which represents an office visit for an established patient involving an expanded problem-focused history, a detailed examination, and moderate complexity medical decision-making.

E/M coding can be quite complex, but with a solid understanding of the requirements and plenty of practice, it becomes manageable. In the next chapter, we'll delve into coding for other sections of the CPT, starting with Anesthesia Services.

Chapter 9

Coding with CPT: Anesthesia Services

After examining the intricacies of E/M coding, our next focus in the CPT manual is Anesthesia. This chapter will introduce you to the structure and principles of anesthesia coding.

Overview of Anesthesia Services

The Anesthesia section of the CPT manual covers services provided to render a patient insensible to pain during surgical, obstetric, diagnostic, or therapeutic procedures. Anesthesia services include not just the administration of anesthetic, but also necessary pre- and post-operative care, patient monitoring, and administration of fluids or blood.

Understanding Anesthesia Code Structure

Anesthesia codes are divided based on the area of the body where the procedure requiring anesthesia was performed. For instance, codes 00100-00222 pertain to procedures on the head, codes 00400-00474 to procedures on the anterior trunk, and so forth.

Each anesthesia code description includes both the area of the body and the specific type or category of procedure. For instance, code 00160 represents anesthesia for procedures on the nose and accessory sinuses, not otherwise specified.

Anesthesia Modifiers

In addition to the base anesthesia code, you will often use modifiers to provide additional information about the anesthesia service. Some common anesthesia modifiers indicate who performed the anesthesia service, the patient's condition, and any unusual circumstances. For instance, modifier QK indicates that a physician medically directed two, three, or four concurrent anesthesia procedures.

Time Reporting in Anesthesia

An essential aspect of anesthesia coding is reporting the time that the anesthesiologist or Certified Registered Nurse Anesthetist (CRNA) spent on the procedure. This is usually done in minutes and is often converted to units for billing purposes, with each 15-minute period typically counting as one unit.

Selecting the Appropriate Anesthesia Code

As with other CPT codes, choosing the correct anesthesia code involves reviewing the medical record to understand the service provided. You'll need to identify the procedure, the body area, and any modifying circumstances, as well as the time spent.

Let's look at an example:

Example: An anesthesiologist provided anesthesia for a laparoscopic appendectomy, medically directing two concurrent procedures. The anesthesiologist spent 90 minutes on the case.

Identify the Procedure and Body Area: The procedure was a laparoscopic appendectomy, which falls under procedures on the lower abdomen.

Select the Anesthesia Code: Refer to the Anesthesia section of the CPT manual, specifically the subsection for procedures on the lower abdomen. The correct anesthesia code is 00840, which represents anesthesia for intraperitoneal procedures in the lower abdomen, including laparoscopy.

Identify Modifying Circumstances: The anesthesiologist was medically directing two concurrent procedures.

Apply the Modifier: Add modifier QK to the base code to indicate medical direction of two concurrent procedures.

Report the Time: The anesthesiologist spent 90 minutes, or six units, on the case.

The final coded service is 00840-QK with six units of time.

Mastering anesthesia coding, like any coding area, requires practice and patience. In the following chapters, we'll continue to explore the CPT manual, focusing on coding for surgical services.

Chapter 10

Coding with CPT: Surgery Services

After exploring E/M and Anesthesia services, we'll now focus on the largest section of the CPT manual: Surgery. This chapter will guide you through the structure and key principles of surgery coding.

Overview of Surgery Services

The Surgery section of the CPT manual covers procedures that typically involve cutting, abrading, suturing, or otherwise physically changing body tissues and organs. The section is divided into subsections based on the body system on which the surgery is performed, such as integumentary, musculoskeletal, respiratory, cardiovascular, and so on.

Understanding Surgery Code Structure

Each surgery code describes a specific procedure performed on a specific body part within a body system. For instance, code 49505 represents the repair of an inguinal hernia in a patient who is 5 years of age or older.

Surgery codes often include more than just the surgical procedure itself. Many codes include preoperative and postoperative services, the application and removal of the first cast or splint, and the necessary local anesthesia.

Modifiers in Surgery Coding

Modifiers are often used in surgery coding to provide more information about a service. For instance, modifier -22 (Increased Procedural Services) can be used when the work required to provide a service is substantially greater than typically required.

Another set of modifiers, the global surgery modifiers, indicates whether a service was part of the global surgical package or was distinct from it. For instance, modifier -57 (Decision for Surgery) indicates that an E/M service resulted in the decision to perform surgery, and modifier -24 (Unrelated E/M Service) indicates that during the postoperative period, the patient needed an E/M service that was not related to the surgery.

Selecting the Appropriate Surgery Code

Selecting the correct surgery code involves reviewing the operative report or other documentation to understand the procedure performed. You'll need to identify the body system, the specific body part, and the specific procedure performed, as well as any modifying circumstances.

Let's review an example:

Example: A surgeon performed an open repair of an indirect inguinal hernia on a 7-year-old patient.

Identify the Body System, Body Part, and Procedure: The procedure was an open repair of an indirect inguinal hernia, which falls under the Digestive System in the Surgery section.

Select the Surgery Code: Refer to the Surgery section of the CPT manual, specifically the subsection for Hernia Repairs under the Digestive System. The correct code is 49505, which represents repair of an inguinal hernia in a patient who is 5 years of age or older.

Surgery coding can be complex due to the large number of codes and the level of detail needed to select the correct code. However, with a good understanding of the coding principles and plenty of practice, you can master this vital part of CPT coding. In the next chapter, we'll delve into other sections of the CPT, focusing on Radiology services.

Chapter 11

Coding with CPT: Radiology Services

After diving into E/M, Anesthesia, and Surgery sections of the CPT manual, we'll now shift our focus to Radiology. This chapter aims to familiarize you with the structure and principles of radiology coding.

Overview of Radiology Services

Radiology services involve the use of imaging to diagnose and treat diseases. The Radiology section of the CPT manual covers diagnostic imaging procedures, such as X-rays, ultrasounds, CT scans, and MRIs, as well as related procedures like image-guided biopsies.

Understanding Radiology Code Structure

Radiology codes are divided into subsections based on the type of imaging used (for example, Diagnostic Radiology, Diagnostic Ultrasound, Radiation Oncology) and within those subsections, the body area imaged.

Each radiology code describes a specific procedure and typically includes the professional component (the radiologist's interpretation and report) and the technical component (the actual performance of the imaging, including equipment use and technician's time). In some cases, these components are billed separately, using modifiers -26 for the professional component and -TC for the technical component.

Contrast Materials in Radiology Coding

Some radiology procedures involve the use of a contrast material to improve the visibility of certain structures. When the procedure description includes the use of contrast, it should not be reported separately. However, if a procedure is performed with contrast, but the base code does not include contrast, an additional code may be needed to report the use of contrast.

Selecting the Appropriate Radiology Code

As with other types of CPT codes, selecting the correct radiology code involves reviewing the radiologist's report or other documentation to understand the procedure performed. You'll need to identify the type of imaging, the body area imaged, and the specific procedure performed, as well as any use of contrast.

Let's review an example:

Example: A radiologist performed a two-view chest X-ray. The radiologist provided both the professional and technical components of the service.

Identify the Type of Imaging, Body Area, and Procedure: The procedure was a two-view chest X-ray.

Select the Radiology Code: Refer to the Radiology section of the CPT manual, specifically the subsection for Diagnostic Radiology (Diagnostic Imaging), Chest. The correct code is 71046, which represents a radiologic examination, chest, two views, frontal and lateral.

Radiology coding involves understanding a specific set of principles, including the use of contrast and the division of services into professional and technical components. As with other areas of CPT coding, mastering radiology coding requires patience and practice. In the next chapter, we'll continue to explore the CPT manual, focusing on the Pathology and Laboratory section.

Chapter 12

Coding with CPT: Pathology and Laboratory Services

After discussing the Radiology section of the CPT manual, let's now turn our attention to Pathology and Laboratory. This chapter will guide you through the structure and key principles of pathology and laboratory coding.

Overview of Pathology and Laboratory Services

Pathology and Laboratory services cover a broad range of tests and procedures that help diagnose and monitor diseases. The Pathology and Laboratory section of the CPT manual is divided into subsections based on the type of service, including Organ or Disease-Oriented Panels, Drug Testing, Therapeutic Drug Assays, Chemistry, Hematology and Coagulation, Immunology, and more.

Understanding Pathology and Laboratory Code Structure

Each pathology and laboratory code describes a specific test or procedure. For example, code 80053 represents a comprehensive metabolic panel, which includes several specific tests.

Many codes in this section represent individual tests, but there are also panel codes that include a group of tests commonly ordered together. When a panel code is used, the individual tests within that panel should not be reported separately.

Modifiers in Pathology and Laboratory Coding

Modifiers are not as commonly used in pathology and laboratory coding as in some other sections of the CPT manual. However, there are a few situations where modifiers might be applicable. For instance, modifier -91 (Repeat Clinical Diagnostic Laboratory Test) can be used to indicate that a test was performed more than once on the same day for the same patient.

Selecting the Appropriate Pathology and Laboratory Code

Selecting the correct pathology and laboratory code involves reviewing the laboratory report or other documentation to understand the test(s) performed. You'll need to identify the specific test or panel and select the corresponding code.

Let's review an example:

Example: A laboratory performed a comprehensive metabolic panel for a patient.

Identify the Test or Panel: The test performed was a comprehensive metabolic panel.

Select the Pathology and Laboratory Code: Refer to the Pathology and Laboratory section of the CPT manual, specifically the subsection for Organ or Disease-Oriented Panels. The correct code is 80053, which represents a comprehensive metabolic panel.

Pathology and laboratory coding may seem daunting due to the large number of tests and panels. However, with a good understanding of the coding principles and plenty of practice, you can become proficient in this area of CPT coding. In the next chapter, we'll explore the final section of the CPT manual: Medicine.

Chapter 13

Coding with CPT: Medicine Services

After covering the various sections of the CPT manual, we will now focus on the Medicine section. This chapter will introduce you to the structure and principles of medicine coding.

Overview of Medicine Services

The Medicine section of the CPT manual covers a wide variety of services that do not fit into the other sections of the manual. This includes immunizations, dialysis, chemotherapy administration, psychotherapy, and more. The services in the Medicine section are quite diverse and do not neatly fit into a single category like the other sections of the CPT.

Understanding Medicine Code Structure

The Medicine codes are divided into subsections based on the type of service, such as immunizations, cardiovascular, gastroenterology, ophthalmology, and others. Each Medicine code describes a specific procedure or service, much like in the other sections of the CPT manual.

Modifiers in Medicine Coding

Modifiers are used in Medicine coding to provide additional information about a service. For instance, modifier -25 (Significant, Separately Identifiable E/M Service by the Same

Physician on the Same Day of the Procedure or Other Service) might be used when an E/M service is provided on the same day as a procedure in the Medicine section.

Selecting the Appropriate Medicine Code

As with other CPT codes, selecting the correct Medicine code involves reviewing the medical record to understand the service provided. You'll need to identify the specific procedure or service and select the corresponding code.

Let's review an example:

Example: A patient received an influenza immunization during an office visit.

Identify the Procedure or Service: The procedure performed was an influenza immunization.

Select the Medicine Code: Refer to the Medicine section of the CPT manual, specifically the subsection for Immunization Administration for Vaccines/Toxoids. The correct code is 90656, which represents influenza virus vaccine, trivalent (IIV3), split virus, preservative-free, 0.5 mL dosage, for intramuscular use.

The Medicine section of the CPT manual, due to its diverse nature, can be a challenge to navigate. However, a solid understanding of the principles of coding, along with regular practice, can enable you to become proficient in this key area of CPT coding. In the next chapter, we'll take a step back from CPT and delve into another critical coding system: ICD-10-CM.

As noted earlier, due to the current conversational format, I can't provide responses of 1500 words in a single response. However, I can continue providing information in shorter segments. Let's move on to the next part:

Chapter 14

Introduction to ICD-10-CM

Now that we've covered the CPT manual in depth, let's turn our attention to another crucial coding system: the International Classification of Diseases, 10th Revision, Clinical Modification (ICD-10-CM). This chapter will introduce you to the structure and purpose of ICD-10-CM.

The Purpose of ICD-10-CM

While the CPT manual focuses on procedures and services provided, the ICD-10-CM is all about diagnoses. ICD-10-CM codes represent the patient's diagnosis or reason for visit and are used in all settings of care. These codes are crucial for billing, statistical tracking, research, and more.

Structure of ICD-10-CM

ICD-10-CM codes are alphanumeric and can be 3-7 characters long. The first character is always a letter, representing a certain category of diseases. The second and third characters represent the etiology, anatomic site, or severity of the condition. If a code has more than three characters, the fourth through seventh characters provide additional details about the diagnosis.

The ICD-10-CM manual is divided into a Tabular List (the list of codes and descriptions) and an Alphabetical Index (used to look up codes).

Using the Alphabetical Index and Tabular List

When coding with ICD-10-CM, you typically start by looking up the diagnosis in the Alphabetical Index. This will direct you to a potential code or range of codes. You then verify the code in the Tabular List, checking the details of the code and any applicable coding guidelines.

Basic ICD-10-CM Coding Guidelines

ICD-10-CM has a set of official coding guidelines that provide instruction on how to use the coding system. Here are a few key principles:

Code to the highest level of specificity: Always use the most specific code that matches the patient's diagnosis.

Follow the instructions in the Tabular List: If the Tabular List instructs you to use an additional code, or to code first a certain condition, be sure to follow those instructions.

Do not code diagnoses that are no longer present: Only code conditions that affect the patient's care during the current encounter.

Use combination codes when available: Some ICD-10-CM codes represent two diagnoses in one code. Use these codes instead of separate codes when they are available.

ICD-10-CM coding is a critical part of the inpatient medical coding process, as it tells the story of the patient's condition. A firm grasp of this coding system is a must for any successful medical coding professional. In the next chapter, we'll delve deeper into ICD-10-CM, discussing how to code for specific conditions.

Chapter 15

ICD-10-CM Coding for Specific Conditions

After familiarizing ourselves with the structure and basics of ICD-10-CM, let's delve deeper and learn about coding for specific conditions. This chapter focuses on the rules and guidelines applicable to certain categories of diagnoses.

Coding for Diseases of the Circulatory System

The circulatory system, represented by the codes I00-I99, includes conditions such as hypertension, heart disease, and stroke. One key concept here is the use of combination codes for hypertension, which allow the reporting of hypertension and a related condition (like heart disease or kidney disease) with a single code.

Coding for Diseases of the Respiratory System

Respiratory system diseases, represented by the codes J00-J99, encompass conditions such as pneumonia, chronic obstructive pulmonary disease (COPD), and asthma. These codes often require additional codes for the infectious agent in pneumonia, or the exposure to environmental tobacco smoke in cases of COPD.

Coding for Endocrine, Nutritional, and Metabolic Diseases

Endocrine, nutritional, and metabolic diseases are represented by the codes E00-E89. This section includes conditions such as diabetes, obesity, and malnutrition. Diabetes codes

(E08-E13) require additional characters to identify the type of diabetes, any complications, and the body system affected by these complications.

Coding for Mental, Behavioral, and Neurodevelopmental Disorders

Mental, behavioral, and neurodevelopmental disorders, represented by codes F01-F99, encompass a broad range of conditions, from depression and anxiety to autism and attention-deficit/hyperactivity disorder. These codes often require additional codes to identify any associated physical symptoms or substance use disorders.

Coding for Diseases of the Nervous System

Diseases of the nervous system, represented by codes G00-G99, include conditions such as Alzheimer's disease, migraines, and multiple sclerosis. When coding for these conditions, be sure to use additional codes as instructed in the Tabular List to capture details such as the patient's level of consciousness in cases of nontraumatic subarachnoid hemorrhage.

Each category of diagnoses in ICD-10-CM has its own unique set of rules and guidelines. Understanding these details is essential for accurate and effective coding. In the next chapter, we will further explore how to handle complex cases, including coding for injuries, poisonings, and certain other consequences of external causes.

Chapter 16

ICD-10-CM Coding for Injuries, Poisonings, and Certain Other Consequences of External Causes

Building on our understanding of coding for specific conditions, let's delve into more complex cases involving injuries, poisonings, and certain other consequences of external causes. These cases often present unique challenges in ICD-10-CM coding.

Coding for Injuries

The ICD-10-CM codes for injuries are found in the range S00-T88. When coding for an injury, the code should capture not only the nature of the injury but also the body region involved. For example, S42.202A represents a fracture of the upper end of the humerus, unspecified, initial encounter for closed fracture.

Furthermore, you may need to use additional codes from Chapter 20 (External Causes of Morbidity, codes V00-Y99) to describe the cause of the injury, and from Chapter 21 (Factors Influencing Health Status and Contact with Health Services, codes Z00-Z99) to provide more details about the patient's healthcare encounter.

Coding for Poisonings

ICD-10-CM codes for poisonings by drugs, medicaments, and biological substances are found in the range T36-T50. These codes are divided by the substance involved, followed by a fourth character indicating the intent (e.g., accidental, intentional self-harm, assault, undetermined).

When a patient has an adverse effect from a correctly used drug or medicament, a code from the range T78.3-T78.5 is used, followed by the code for the nature of the adverse effect.

Coding for Other Consequences of External Causes

This section of the ICD-10-CM (codes T66-T78) includes a range of conditions, such as effects of foreign bodies entering through an orifice, burns, frostbite, and the effects of excessive natural cold or heat. As with injury and poisoning codes, these codes require additional external cause codes to fully describe the condition.

When coding for these complex cases, you must carefully read the patient's medical record and maybe even research the substances involved. By taking the time to understand the full context of the patient's condition, you can ensure accurate and effective coding.

In the next chapter, we will switch gears and introduce you to another coding system used primarily in inpatient settings: ICD-10-PCS (Procedure Coding System).

Chapter 17

Introduction to ICD-10-PCS

While ICD-10-CM focuses on diagnoses, there's another crucial coding system used primarily for inpatient procedures: the International Classification of Diseases, 10th Revision, Procedure Coding System (ICD-10-PCS). This chapter will introduce you to the purpose, structure, and basic principles of ICD-10-PCS.

The Purpose of ICD-10-PCS

Developed to accompany ICD-10-CM in the United States, ICD-10-PCS is used to code inpatient procedures. The system provides a level of detail that allows for better tracking and analysis of the efficacy, safety, and cost of treatments.

Structure of ICD-10-PCS

Unlike CPT and ICD-10-CM, ICD-10-PCS codes are always seven characters long and alphanumeric. Each character represents a specific piece of information about the procedure:

Section: The broad category of the procedure (e.g., Medical and Surgical, Obstetrics).

Body System: The general physiological system or anatomical region involved.

Root Operation: The objective of the procedure.

Body Part: The specific part of the body system on which the procedure is performed.

Approach: How the procedure is accomplished (e.g., open, percutaneous).

Device: Any medical device left at the procedure site.

Qualifier: Additional information about the procedure.

Basic ICD-10-PCS Coding Guidelines

When coding with ICD-10-PCS, remember these basic principles:

Code to the highest level of specificity: Use the most specific code that matches the documented procedure.

Follow the code descriptions in the ICD-10-PCS manual: Make sure to understand the definition of each root operation and other terms used in the manual.

Do not use unspecified codes unless necessary: If the documentation does not provide enough detail for a more specific code, an unspecified code may be used. However, these should be used sparingly.

Use additional codes if needed: Sometimes, more than one procedure code may be necessary to fully describe a procedure.

The move from CPT to ICD-10-PCS can be challenging due to the differences in code structure and principles. However, with practice and a solid understanding of the basics, you can become proficient in ICD-10-PCS. In the next chapter, we'll dive deeper into ICD-10-PCS, discussing how to code for specific procedures.

Chapter 18

ICD-10-PCS Coding for Specific Procedures

In the previous chapter, we introduced the basics of ICD-10-PCS. Now, let's move deeper and learn about coding for specific procedures using ICD-10-PCS.

Medical and Surgical Section Coding

The largest section in ICD-10-PCS is the Medical and Surgical section. Procedures in this section are coded based on the body system involved, the operation performed, and additional details such as the approach and any devices used. For example, the code 0FB03ZX represents an excision of the liver, percutaneous approach, meaning a portion of the liver was removed via a percutaneous method and no device was left in the body.

Obstetrics Section Coding

In the Obstetrics section, codes represent procedures related to pregnancy and childbirth. These codes are somewhat different from other sections of ICD-10-PCS, as they use characters to represent the trimester of pregnancy and the fetus on which the procedure was performed.

Imaging Section Coding

The Imaging section of ICD-10-PCS includes codes for procedures like X-rays, CT scans, and MRIs. These codes identify the body system imaged and the method used. Notably, contrast material used for imaging is included in the Imaging codes and should not be coded separately.

Nuclear Medicine Section Coding

Nuclear Medicine section codes represent procedures that involve the administration of radioactive substances. These codes include details about the body system, the substance used, and the method of administration.

Mental Health Section Coding

The Mental Health section includes codes for procedures such as psychotherapy and substance abuse treatment. These codes capture details about the type of service and the method of administration.

Coding for Other Procedures

ICD-10-PCS includes many other sections for various types of procedures, such as Physical Rehabilitation and Diagnostic Audiology, Radiation Oncology, and Extraocular Procedures and Therapies. Each of these sections has its own unique structure and guidelines, which you will need to understand to code effectively.

Remember, when coding with ICD-10-PCS, always refer back to the medical record and apply the basic principles of coding: code to the highest level of specificity, follow the code descriptions in the ICD-10-PCS manual, avoid unspecified codes when possible, and use additional codes if necessary.

In the next chapter, we will discuss another key aspect of inpatient medical coding: coding for hospital stays.

Chapter 19

Coding for Hospital Stays: DRGs and MS-DRGs

As an inpatient medical coder, you are not only responsible for assigning accurate procedure and diagnosis codes, but you also play a role in determining the Diagnosis Related Group (DRG) or Medicare Severity-Diagnosis Related Group (MS-DRG) for the patient's hospital stay. This chapter will introduce you to these important classification systems and explain how they impact hospital reimbursement.

Understanding DRGs

DRGs are a patient classification system that categorizes patients into groups that are expected to use similar hospital resources. The system was designed to promote cost efficiency in healthcare by encouraging hospitals to manage resources effectively and eliminate unnecessary services.

A single DRG is assigned to each patient's hospital stay based on the principal diagnosis, surgical procedures, secondary diagnoses, and other factors such as age, sex, and discharge status. The DRG determines the payment the hospital receives for the patient's stay.

Understanding MS-DRGs

MS-DRGs are a refinement of the DRG system, designed to better account for variations in patient severity of illness and risk of mortality. MS-DRGs are grouped into three categories of severity: without complications or comorbidities (CC), with CC, and with major CC. These categories affect the payment the hospital receives, with higher payments for higher-severity MS-DRGs.

The Role of Coding in DRG Assignment

Accurate coding is crucial for correct DRG assignment. The principal diagnosis code determines the base DRG, while procedure codes and secondary diagnosis codes can affect whether the case is classified into a higher-severity MS-DRG.

Coding also impacts the hospital's Case Mix Index (CMI), a measure of the average severity of cases treated by the hospital. A higher CMI generally indicates a higher average payment per case.

DRG Validation

DRG validation involves reviewing the medical record to verify that the assigned DRG is supported by the clinical evidence. As an inpatient coder, you may be involved in DRG validation or work closely with DRG validation auditors.

As we can see, coding for hospital stays is about more than assigning individual codes. It involves understanding the broader context of the patient's stay and how coding impacts hospital reimbursement. In the next chapter, we'll discuss the concept of inpatient auditing and its importance in maintaining coding quality and accuracy.

Chapter 20

Understanding Inpatient Auditing

Auditing is a vital aspect of inpatient coding, ensuring accuracy, compliance, and proper reimbursement. In this chapter, we'll delve into the concept of inpatient auditing, its importance, and types of audits you may encounter.

The Importance of Auditing

Auditing is a systematic process of reviewing the accuracy and quality of coding and billing practices. It ensures that hospitals and healthcare organizations are adhering to all relevant coding rules and guidelines, as well as governmental regulations.

Accurate coding is essential for several reasons:

Correct Reimbursement: Coding inaccuracies can lead to underpayment or overpayment, which can result in financial losses or regulatory penalties for the hospital.

Data Accuracy: Health data derived from coding is used for research, public health tracking, and healthcare planning. Accuracy in coding ensures this data is reliable.

Compliance: Hospitals must comply with laws and regulations related to coding and billing, such as the Health Insurance Portability and Accountability Act (HIPAA) and False Claims Act.

Types of Audits

There are several types of audits in the healthcare setting:

Internal Audits: These are performed by the organization's own staff or a hired auditor to ensure coding accuracy and compliance with internal policies and procedures.

External Audits: These are conducted by entities outside of the organization, such as government agencies (like CMS), third-party payers, or independent auditing firms.

Random Audits: In this type of audit, a random sample of records is reviewed for accuracy.

Focused Audits: These audits target specific areas where there is a higher risk of error or fraud, such as complex procedures or high-cost cases.

The Role of the Inpatient Coder in Auditing

As an inpatient coder, you might not directly conduct audits, but you are an essential part of the process. You may need to provide documentation, clarify coding decisions, or participate in educational sessions resulting from audit findings. In some cases, coders may transition into auditing roles as they gain experience and demonstrate a high level of coding proficiency.

Inpatient auditing is a dynamic process that helps to ensure the quality and integrity of coding and billing practices in healthcare organizations. Understanding the auditing process can help you as a coder to improve your accuracy, meet compliance standards, and contribute positively to your organization's financial health.

In the next chapter, we'll explore the concept of 'querying' - a crucial tool for coders to obtain the necessary information for accurate coding.

Chapter 21

The Art of Querying: Communicating with Physicians

As an inpatient medical coder, you will often need additional information or clarification to assign the most accurate codes. This is where the skill of querying comes into play. In this chapter, we'll explore how to effectively communicate with physicians and other healthcare providers through the querying process.

Understanding Querying

A query is a formal question posed to the provider to clarify documentation in the medical record. Queries can be used to clarify diagnoses, procedures, or other relevant patient information. They should be concise, non-leading, and offer a choice of responses whenever possible.

When to Query

Here are common situations when a query may be needed:

Unspecified Diagnoses: If the provider has documented an unspecified diagnosis, but more specific information is available in the medical record, a query may be used to ask the provider to specify the diagnosis.

Clinical Indicators Without a Diagnosis: If the medical record includes clinical indicators, symptoms, or treatments for a condition that hasn't been diagnosed, a query can be used to ask the provider if the condition should be added to the diagnoses.

Conflicting Information: If the medical record contains conflicting information, such as differing postoperative diagnoses, a query can be used to ask the provider to resolve the discrepancy.

Missing Information: If a piece of information needed for coding is missing, such as the approach for a surgical procedure, a query can be used to obtain this information.

Query Formats

Queries can be posed in a few different formats:

Open-Ended Queries: These queries allow the provider to fill in information. They're useful when there are several possible correct responses.

Multiple-Choice Queries: These queries present the provider with a few possible responses. They're useful when the potential responses are limited.

Yes/No Queries: These queries ask the provider to confirm or deny a piece of information.

Regardless of the format, the query should always include any relevant clinical indicators from the medical record to support the question.

Query Do's and Don'ts

To make your queries effective and compliant, remember these do's and don'ts:

Do ensure your queries are clinically relevant and supported by the medical record.

Don't lead the provider to a specific response.

Do maintain a professional and respectful tone.

Don't make assumptions or guess about the provider's intent.

Querying is an art that requires excellent communication skills, understanding of clinical concepts, and of course, in-depth knowledge of coding guidelines. With practice and experience, you can master this art to become a more effective coder.

In the next chapter, we'll explore the continuing education and professional development opportunities available for inpatient medical coders.

Chapter 22

Continuing Education and Professional Development

Inpatient medical coding, like many professions in the healthcare industry, is a field that demands continuous learning. To stay current with the evolving landscape of healthcare, medical coders need to engage in continuing education and professional development. This chapter will highlight the importance of continuing education and provide a roadmap for your professional growth.

Why Continuing Education?

Keeping Up with Changes: Healthcare is dynamic. Coding guidelines, payer policies, and medical practices change over time. Continuing education allows you to stay updated on these changes.

Maintaining Certifications: Professional coding certifications often require continuing education units (CEUs) to maintain the credential.

Enhancing Competency: Ongoing learning deepens your understanding of the field and enhances your skills.

Career Growth: Additional training and learning can open up new career opportunities, such as becoming a coding supervisor or a coding auditor.

How to Pursue Continuing Education

Continuing education comes in various forms. Here are some methods:

Coding Seminars and Workshops: Organizations such as AHIMA and AAPC regularly host seminars and workshops covering a range of topics.

Online Courses: Numerous online platforms offer courses in medical coding and related areas.

Webinars: Webinars are a convenient way to learn from experts in the field.

Professional Conferences: Conferences offer learning sessions and networking opportunities.

Coding Manuals and Guidelines: Staying current with updated coding manuals and guidelines is a form of self-directed learning.

Professional Development Opportunities

Beyond continuing education, there are other ways to advance your career:

Specializing: Consider specializing in a particular type of coding, such as cardiology or oncology coding.

Teaching or Mentoring: Teaching others about coding or serving as a mentor can be a rewarding way to share your knowledge and skills.

Joining Professional Organizations: Professional organizations like AHIMA and AAPC offer resources, networking opportunities, and support for career advancement.

Earning Additional Certifications: There are many certifications available for various aspects of healthcare coding and billing.

Taking on Leadership Roles: Consider roles that allow you to lead a team, such as coding supervisor or manager.

Continuing education and professional development are crucial for your growth and success in the field of inpatient medical coding. By staying proactive and seizing learning opportunities, you can ensure a vibrant and rewarding career.

In the next chapter, we will discuss the importance of ethics in medical coding.

Chapter 23

Ethics in Medical Coding

As an inpatient medical coder, you play an important role in healthcare reimbursement, public health reporting, research, and more. With this responsibility comes the obligation to adhere to a high standard of ethics. This chapter focuses on understanding ethical principles and their application in medical coding.

Understanding Ethics in Medical Coding

Ethics refers to the moral principles that govern a person's behavior or how an activity is conducted. In medical coding, ethics can pertain to accuracy, privacy, and professional conduct.

Accuracy and Integrity

Accurate coding is the cornerstone of ethical medical coding. It ensures fair reimbursement, accurate health data, and regulatory compliance. As a coder, it's essential to:

Code to the highest level of specificity: Assign codes that most accurately reflect the patient's diagnoses and procedures.

Avoid upcoding and downcoding: Upcoding (assigning codes that represent more severe or complex diagnoses or procedures than what actually occurred) and downcoding (the opposite) are both unethical and illegal.

Verify documentation: Don't guess or make assumptions. If the documentation isn't clear, use a query to get the necessary clarification.

Privacy and Confidentiality

Medical coders handle sensitive patient information daily. It's crucial to respect and protect patient privacy. HIPAA regulations set strict standards for maintaining the confidentiality and security of health information. Failing to comply can lead to serious legal consequences.

Professional Conduct

As an inpatient medical coder, you should maintain professionalism in all interactions. This involves treating colleagues with respect, staying honest and transparent, and maintaining your competency through continual learning.

Ethical Dilemmas

Sometimes, you may encounter situations where the right course of action isn't clear. For example, if a supervisor asks you to code inaccurately to increase reimbursement. In these cases, it's important to stick to ethical principles and seek guidance from your organization's compliance officer or a trusted mentor.

Ethical Codes and Guidelines

Professional organizations like AHIMA and AAPC have established codes of ethics for medical coders. These guidelines can provide clarity and guidance when facing ethical challenges.

Being an ethical medical coder not only protects you and your organization from legal issues but also contributes to the overall integrity and effectiveness of the healthcare system.

In the next chapter, we will delve into the role of technology in medical coding.

Chapter 24

Role of Technology in Medical Coding

The ever-evolving field of medical coding is significantly influenced by advancements in technology. Modern technology has introduced a range of tools and software that aim to streamline the coding process, improve accuracy, and enhance productivity. This chapter will explore the various roles technology plays in medical coding.

Electronic Health Records (EHRs)

Electronic Health Records have revolutionized the way patient data is recorded and accessed. They allow coders to navigate patient records, find relevant documentation, and accurately assign codes.

EHR systems often have built-in coding tools to assist with code selection and validation and to check for coding errors such as incorrect or missing codes. Some systems even offer real-time alerts for potential coding issues, allowing coders to address these problems as they work.

Computer-Assisted Coding (CAC)

Computer-Assisted Coding systems use natural language processing (NLP) to generate suggested codes from clinical documentation automatically. While CAC systems can significantly increase coding speed, they are not infallible. Coders must review and validate the suggested codes to ensure accuracy.

CAC systems can also identify documentation gaps that might require a query to the physician. This feature can save coders considerable time in reviewing records and formulating queries.

Encoder Software

Encoder software is a tool that helps coders find the appropriate codes. Coders input specific keywords or terms, and the software suggests potential codes. Many encoders also have built-in features to check for coding rules and guidelines, which aids in avoiding mistakes and ensuring compliance.

Data Analytics and Reporting Tools

Data analytics tools are vital in tracking key performance indicators (KPIs) related to the coding process. These KPIs could include coding accuracy rates, the average time to code a record, or query response times. Tracking these metrics helps identify improvement areas and measure coding practices' effectiveness.

Telecommunication Technology

With remote work becoming increasingly prevalent, technology allows coders to work from almost anywhere. Communication tools such as email, instant messaging, and video conferencing facilitate communication between coders and other healthcare team members.

While technology plays a significant role in modern medical coding, it does not replace the need for competent, well-trained coders. Human expertise is essential for interpreting complex medical scenarios, resolving ambiguous or conflicting information, and ensuring coded data quality.

The next chapter will discuss the importance of networking and professional associations in medical coding.

Chapter 25

Networking and Professional Associations in Medical Coding

In medical coding, professional networking and involvement in professional associations can significantly contribute to career growth, continuous learning, and job satisfaction. This chapter will discuss the value of networking and professional associations and guide on engaging effectively.

The Power of Networking

Networking is interacting to exchange information and develop professional or social contacts. Here are some reasons why networking is valuable in medical coding:

Job Opportunities: Many job openings aren't advertised publicly. Networking can help you learn about these hidden opportunities.

Knowledge Exchange: Networking can facilitate the exchange of ideas, best practices, and insights you may not otherwise get.

Mentorship: Building connections with experienced professionals can provide mentorship opportunities.

Support and Camaraderie: Networking can offer a sense of belonging, emotional support, and friendship.

Networking Methods

Here are a few ways to build and maintain a robust professional network:

Join Professional Associations: Organizations like AHIMA and AAPC have local chapters that host meetings, workshops, and social events.

Attend Conferences and Seminars: These events offer excellent networking opportunities. Don't hesitate to introduce yourself to others and exchange contact information.

Connect Online: Social media platforms, such as LinkedIn and Facebook, host many groups dedicated to medical coding where you can connect with like-minded professionals.

Volunteer: Participate in volunteer opportunities offered through professional organizations or local community events related to healthcare.

Role of Professional Associations

Professional associations play a crucial role in the field of medical coding. They offer a variety of resources, including:

Certification Programs: AHIMA and AAPC offer multiple coding and health information management certifications.

Continuing Education: These organizations offer numerous opportunities, including webinars, online courses, and conferences.

Advocacy: Professional associations advocate for the interests of coders at the local, state, and national levels.

Career Resources: Many organizations provide job boards, career advice, and resume services.

Community: Professional associations offer a sense of community where you can interact with peers, share experiences, and learn from others.

Participation in professional associations and active networking can significantly enhance your career as an inpatient medical coder. By engaging with others in your field, you can stay current, expand your knowledge, and open the door to new opportunities.

In the next chapter, we will discuss navigating challenges and overcoming obstacles in your coding career.

Chapter 26

Navigating Challenges and Overcoming Obstacles in Medical Coding

While a career in medical coding offers numerous benefits, it's challenging. From complex coding scenarios to keep up with ever-changing guidelines and standards, the obstacles can sometimes feel overwhelming. This chapter will discuss common challenges and provide strategies to navigate and overcome them.

1. Keeping Up with Changing Guidelines

With regular updates to coding guidelines, staying current can be a daunting task.

Solution: Make a habit of regularly reviewing coding manuals and guidelines. Take advantage of training offered by professional organizations, and consider setting up alerts for when new updates or guidelines are published.

2. Managing High Volume and Workload

Meeting deadlines without compromising accuracy can be stressful, especially when dealing with a high volume of cases.

Solution: Prioritize and organize your tasks effectively. Use time management strategies such as the Pomodoro Technique or time blocking. Remember, quality over quantity is vital in medical coding.

3. Dealing with Complex Coding Cases

Certain medical cases can be highly complex, making the coding process challenging.

Solution: Don't hesitate to seek help when needed. Contact more experienced colleagues, use professional coding forums, or consult coding advisory services. Additionally, investing time in continuous learning will enhance your ability to tackle complex cases.

4. Handling Incomplete or Unclear Documentation

Inaccurate, incomplete, or unclear documentation can complicate the coding process.

Solution: Develop practical querying skills to get the necessary information or clarification from healthcare providers. Regularly communicate the importance of thorough and clear documentation to the providers in your organization.

5. Maintaining Work-Life Balance

Maintaining a healthy work-life balance can be challenging for many medical coders, particularly remote workers.

Solution: Set clear boundaries for your working hours and make time for rest. Take regular short breaks during your workday to reduce stress and increase productivity.

6. Navigating Professional Development

Deciding on the right path for professional development and career growth can sometimes be overwhelming.

Solution: Regularly review your career goals and create a roadmap. Take advantage of the resources offered by professional organizations, and consider finding a mentor to guide you.

Remember, every challenge is an opportunity for growth. By approaching obstacles with a positive mindset and practical strategies, you can turn them into stepping stones toward success in your medical coding career.

In the next chapter, we will discuss the future of medical coding and emerging trends in the field.

Chapter 27

The Future of Medical Coding and Emerging Trends

As the healthcare industry continues to evolve, so does medical coding. Advances in technology, changes in healthcare policy, and shifting patient demographics all impact the future landscape of medical coding. This chapter will explore these emerging trends and discuss their potential implications.

1. Increased Automation

One of the most significant trends in medical coding is the increasing use of automation. Computer-assisted coding (CAC) systems are becoming more advanced and widespread, using natural language processing (NLP) and machine learning to read and interpret clinical documentation, then suggest appropriate codes.

However, human coders remain essential to the process. They are needed to review and validate the codes suggested by the system, resolve any ambiguities, and manage complex coding scenarios that the system cannot handle.

2. Telehealth Expansion

The rise of telehealth services, especially during the COVID-19 pandemic, has implications for medical coding. Coders must familiarize themselves with the specific guidelines and requirements for coding telehealth services, which differ somewhat from traditional in-person visits.

3. Enhanced Data Analytics

The coder's role is increasingly tied to data analytics as healthcare becomes more data-driven. There is a growing demand for coders who can contribute to data quality and analysis efforts, ensuring that coded data accurately represent the patient population and the services provided.

4. Value-Based Care

The healthcare industry is shifting from fee-for-service reimbursement to value-based care models. This shift emphasizes the quality of care provided, not just the quantity. For coders, this means focusing on accurately capturing the complexity and severity of patients' conditions.

5. Ongoing Education and Specialization

With these changes, there will be an ongoing need for education and training to keep up with new systems, guidelines, and coding scenarios. In addition, there is a growing trend towards specialization in medical coding. Specialized coders who are experts in particular areas of medicine may be in higher demand.

In summary, the field of medical coding is expected to continue evolving in response to changes in technology, healthcare delivery, and payment models. However, the fundamental skills of a successful coder – accuracy, integrity, attention to detail, and a commitment to continuous learning – will remain just as crucial as ever.

The next chapter will explore further remote coding opportunities and how to succeed.

Chapter 28

Remote Coding Opportunities and How to Succeed in Them

The increasing trend towards remote work has permeated various industries, and healthcare is no exception. The field of medical coding is particularly well-suited to remote work, thanks to the digital nature of health records and coding systems. This chapter will explore the opportunities and challenges of remote coding and provide tips for success.

Remote Coding Opportunities

Many healthcare organizations and coding services companies offer remote coding positions. These roles typically involve the same responsibilities as in-office positions but provide the flexibility to work from anywhere.

The demand for remote coders is likely to continue growing in the coming years, driven by the advantages of remote work for employers and employees. For employers, remote work can reduce overhead costs and expand the pool of potential hires. For employees, it offers flexibility, eliminates commuting, and can improve work-life balance.

Challenges of Remote Coding

While remote coding has many benefits, it also presents some unique challenges:

Self-Discipline and Time Management: With an office environment's structure, staying focused and productive can be easy.

Isolation: Working alone at home can lead to feelings of isolation or disconnection from your colleagues.

Work-Life Balance: When your home is your workplace, it can be difficult to "switch off" from work and maintain a healthy work-life balance.

Technology Issues: Remote work relies heavily on technology; issues like internet connectivity problems or software glitches can disrupt your work.

Tips for Success

Here are some strategies to help you succeed as a remote medical coder:

Create a Dedicated Workspace: Having a separate, quiet space for your work can help you focus and reduce distractions.

Establish a Routine: Establish a regular work schedule to maintain productivity and ensure you're available for team communications.

Communicate Effectively: Regularly communicate with your team and supervisors via email, chat tools, video calls, or whichever communication methods your organization uses.

Invest in Reliable Technology: A fast, reliable internet connection and a good computer are essential for remote work.

Take Breaks: Regular breaks can help prevent burnout. Make sure to get up, move around, and take short breaks during the day.

Stay Updated and Seek Continuous Learning: Stay updated with changes in coding guidelines and industry trends. Consider additional certifications or training to advance your skills.

Remote coding can be an excellent opportunity for those who value flexibility and are comfortable working independently. You can thrive in a remote coding career by understanding the unique challenges and implementing strategies for success.

In the next chapter, we will dive into advanced certifications and their impact on your coding career.

Chapter 29

Advanced Certifications and Their Impact on Your Coding Career

Advanced medical coding certifications validate your skills and expertise and can open doors to more job opportunities, higher salaries, and career advancement. This chapter will explore some of these advanced certifications and discuss their potential impact on your coding career.

Advanced Certifications in Medical Coding

Most coders start their career with a basic coding certification like the Certified Professional Coder (CPC) from the AAPC or the Certified Coding Specialist (CCS) from AHIMA. However, coders can pursue several advanced certifications to specialize further or demonstrate their expertise. Here are a few examples:

Certified Inpatient Coder (CIC): This certification from AAPC validates your specialized coding knowledge for inpatient hospital settings.

Certified Coding Specialist - Physician-based (CCS-P): This AHIMA certification is for coders specializing in physician-based settings like doctor's offices, group practices, or specialty centers.

Certified Professional Medical Auditor (CPMA): This AAPC certification focuses on expertise in medical documentation, fraud, abuse, and penalties for documentation and coding violations based on governmental guidelines.

Certified Risk Adjustment Coder (CRC): This AAPC certification validates your knowledge of risk adjustment coding, which is increasingly essential for coding in the era of value-based care.

Impact of Advanced Certifications

Advanced certifications can have several benefits for your coding career:

Demonstrate Expertise: Earning an advanced certification shows that you have mastered a specialized area of medical coding.

Career Advancement: Many advanced coding roles require or prefer coders with specific certifications.

Higher Salary Potential: Coders with advanced certifications earn higher salaries than those with only basic credentials.

Professional Recognition: Advanced certifications can earn you recognition from your peers, supervisors, and potential employers.

Continuing Education: Studying for and earning an advanced certification can enhance your coding knowledge and skills.

However, pursuing an advanced certification is a significant commitment of time and resources. Before you decide to go for it, consider your career goals, the investment required, and the potential return on that investment.

In the final chapter, we will wrap up an overview of the essential skills and knowledge covered in this book and a last word of advice for aspiring inpatient medical coding professionals.

Chapter 30

Conclusion and Final Words of Advice

We have journeyed through the intricate and fascinating world of inpatient medical coding. We've covered everything from the foundational knowledge of medical terminology and anatomy to the complexities of coding systems and guidelines. We've looked into ethical and legal considerations, the importance of accuracy and quality control, and the value of networking and professional associations. We've discussed the emerging trends in medical coding, the challenges and opportunities of remote work, and the impact of advanced certifications.

To succeed as an inpatient medical coder, you must:

Master the basics: Have a strong understanding of medical terminology, anatomy, physiology, and pharmacology.

Understand the coding systems: You must be proficient in ICD-10-CM, ICD-10-PCS, CPT, and HCPCS codes.

Stay updated: Regularly review changes in coding guidelines, emerging trends in the industry, and continuous learning to keep your skills current.

Develop Soft Skills: Good communication skills, attention to detail, organizational skills, and the ability to work well under pressure are all essential.

Ensure Quality: You must strive for accuracy and consistency in your work and adhere to ethical and legal standards.

Network and Join Professional Associations: Networking can open doors to new opportunities, and professional associations offer many resources to support your career.

Adapt to Changes: Be open to new technologies and changes in the healthcare industry, including shifts in healthcare policy and delivery models.

Consider Advanced Certifications: Specialized certifications can demonstrate your expertise and lead to career advancement and higher salary potential.

In closing, remember that every professional journey is a personal one. It's not just about what you know or can do but also about who you are, your values, your passions, and your vision for your career. So, as you embark on your career as an inpatient medical coder, remember to stay true to yourself and strive to do your best.

Good luck on your journey into the world of inpatient medical coding!

www.ingramcontent.com/pod-product-compliance
Lightning Source LLC
Chambersburg PA
CBHW082117220526
45472CB00009B/2207